This book belongs to:

Restaurant:

Date:

Time:

Occasion: ❑ Date Night   ❑ Birthday
            ❑

In the company of:

Server name:

Warm welcome: ❑ Yes   ❑ Average   ❑ No
Quick service: ❑ Yes   ❑ Average   ❑ Poor
Accuracy: ❑ Good   ❑ Average   ❑ Poor

Ambiance: ❑ Beautiful   ❑ Romantic
            ❑ Average   ❑ Disappointing

Cleanliness Restrooms: ❑ Good   ❑ Average   ❑ Poor
Cleanliness overall: ❑ Good   ❑ Average   ❑ Poor

Drinks ordered: Meals ordered:

Quality overall: ❑ Good   ❑ Average   ❑ Poor

Value for Money: ❑ Overpriced   ❑ OK   ❑ Great

Shall we go again?   ❑ Yes   ❑ No

Memories

Restaurant:
Date:
Time:

Occasion: ❑ Date Night ❑ Birthday
❑

In the company of:

Server name:

Warm welcome: ❑ Yes ❑ Average ❑ No
Quick service: ❑ Yes ❑ Average ❑ Poor
Accuracy: ❑ Good ❑ Average ❑ Poor

Ambiance: ❑ Beautiful ❑ Romantic
❑ Average ❑ Disappointing

Cleanliness Restrooms: ❑ Good ❑ Average ❑ Poor
Cleanliness overall: ❑ Good ❑ Average ❑ Poor

Drinks ordered: Meals ordered:

Quality overall: ❑ Good ❑ Average ❑ Poor

Value for Money: ❑ Overpriced ❑ OK ❑ Great

Shall we go again? ❑ Yes ❑ No

Memories

Restaurant:

Date:

Time:

Occasion: ❑ Date Night ❑ Birthday
❑

In the company of:

Server name:

Warm welcome: ❑ Yes ❑ Average ❑ No
Quick service: ❑ Yes ❑ Average ❑ Poor
Accuracy: ❑ Good ❑ Average ❑ Poor

Ambiance: ❑ Beautiful ❑ Romantic
❑ Average ❑ Disappointing

Cleanliness Restrooms: ❑ Good ❑ Average ❑ Poor
Cleanliness overall: ❑ Good ❑ Average ❑ Poor

Drinks ordered: Meals ordered:

Quality overall: ❑ Good ❑ Average ❑ Poor

Value for Money: ❑ Overpriced ❑ OK ❑ Great

Shall we go again? ❑ Yes ❑ No

Memories

Restaurant:
Date:
Time:

Occasion: ❑ Date Night ❑ Birthday
❑

In the company of:

Server name:

Warm welcome: ❑ Yes ❑ Average ❑ No
Quick service: ❑ Yes ❑ Average ❑ Poor
Accuracy: ❑ Good ❑ Average ❑ Poor

Ambiance: ❑ Beautiful ❑ Romantic
❑ Average ❑ Disappointing

Cleanliness Restrooms: ❑ Good ❑ Average ❑ Poor
Cleanliness overall: ❑ Good ❑ Average ❑ Poor

Drinks ordered: Meals ordered:

Quality overall: ❑ Good ❑ Average ❑ Poor

Value for Money: ❑ Overpriced ❑ OK ❑ Great

Shall we go again? ❑ Yes ❑ No

Memories

Restaurant:
Date:
Time:

Occasion: ☐ Date Night   ☐ Birthday
           ☐

In the company of:

Server name:

Warm welcome: ☐ Yes   ☐ Average   ☐ No
Quick service: ☐ Yes   ☐ Average   ☐ Poor
Accuracy: ☐ Good   ☐ Average   ☐ Poor

Ambiance: ☐ Beautiful   ☐ Romantic
           ☐ Average   ☐ Disappointing

Cleanliness Restrooms: ☐ Good   ☐ Average   ☐ Poor
Cleanliness overall: ☐ Good   ☐ Average   ☐ Poor

Drinks ordered: Meals ordered:

Quality overall: ☐ Good   ☐ Average   ☐ Poor

Value for Money: ☐ Overpriced   ☐ OK   ☐ Great

Shall we go again?   ☐ Yes   ☐ No

Memories

Restaurant:

Date:

Time:

Occasion: ❑ Date Night   ❑ Birthday
           ❑

In the company of:

Server name:

Warm welcome: ❑ Yes   ❑ Average   ❑ No
Quick service: ❑ Yes   ❑ Average   ❑ Poor
Accuracy: ❑ Good   ❑ Average   ❑ Poor

Ambiance: ❑ Beautiful   ❑ Romantic
           ❑ Average   ❑ Disappointing

Cleanliness Restrooms: ❑ Good   ❑ Average   ❑ Poor
Cleanliness overall: ❑ Good   ❑ Average   ❑ Poor

Drinks ordered: Meals ordered:

Quality overall: ❑ Good   ❑ Average   ❑ Poor

Value for Money: ❑ Overpriced   ❑ OK   ❑ Great

Shall we go again?   ❑ Yes   ❑ No

Memories

Restaurant:
Date:
Time:

Occasion: ❑ Date Night ❑ Birthday
❑

In the company of:

Server name:

Warm welcome: ❑ Yes ❑ Average ❑ No
Quick service: ❑ Yes ❑ Average ❑ Poor
Accuracy: ❑ Good ❑ Average ❑ Poor

Ambiance: ❑ Beautiful ❑ Romantic
❑ Average ❑ Disappointing

Cleanliness Restrooms: ❑ Good ❑ Average ❑ Poor
Cleanliness overall: ❑ Good ❑ Average ❑ Poor

Drinks ordered: Meals ordered:

Quality overall: ❑ Good ❑ Average ❑ Poor

Value for Money: ❑ Overpriced ❑ OK ❑ Great

Shall we go again? ❑ Yes ❑ No

Memories

Restaurant:
Date:
Time:

Occasion: ☐ Date Night ☐ Birthday
☐

In the company of:

Server name:

Warm welcome: ☐ Yes ☐ Average ☐ No
Quick service: ☐ Yes ☐ Average ☐ Poor
Accuracy: ☐ Good ☐ Average ☐ Poor

Ambiance: ☐ Beautiful ☐ Romantic
☐ Average ☐ Disappointing

Cleanliness Restrooms: ☐ Good ☐ Average ☐ Poor
Cleanliness overall: ☐ Good ☐ Average ☐ Poor

Drinks ordered: Meals ordered:

Quality overall: ☐ Good ☐ Average ☐ Poor

Value for Money: ☐ Overpriced ☐ OK ☐ Great

Shall we go again? ☐ Yes ☐ No

Memories

Restaurant:
Date:
Time:

Occasion: ❑ Date Night   ❑ Birthday
           ❑

In the company of:

Server name:

Warm welcome: ❑ Yes   ❑ Average   ❑ No
Quick service: ❑ Yes   ❑ Average   ❑ Poor
Accuracy: ❑ Good   ❑ Average   ❑ Poor

Ambiance: ❑ Beautiful   ❑ Romantic
                 ❑ Average   ❑ Disappointing

Cleanliness Restrooms: ❑ Good   ❑ Average   ❑ Poor
Cleanliness overall: ❑ Good   ❑ Average   ❑ Poor

Drinks ordered: Meals ordered:

Quality overall: ❑ Good   ❑ Average   ❑ Poor

Value for Money: ❑ Overpriced   ❑ OK   ❑ Great

Shall we go again?   ❑ Yes   ❑ No

Memories

Restaurant:
Date:
Time:

Occasion: ❑ Date Night ❑ Birthday
❑

In the company of:

Server name:

Warm welcome: ❑ Yes ❑ Average ❑ No
Quick service: ❑ Yes ❑ Average ❑ Poor
Accuracy: ❑ Good ❑ Average ❑ Poor

Ambiance: ❑ Beautiful ❑ Romantic
❑ Average ❑ Disappointing

Cleanliness Restrooms: ❑ Good ❑ Average ❑ Poor
Cleanliness overall: ❑ Good ❑ Average ❑ Poor

Drinks ordered: Meals ordered:

Quality overall: ❑ Good ❑ Average ❑ Poor

Value for Money: ❑ Overpriced ❑ OK ❑ Great

Shall we go again? ❑ Yes ❑ No

Memories

Restaurant:
Date:
Time:

Occasion:
    ❑ Date Night   ❑ Birthday
    ❑

In the company of:

Server name:

Warm welcome: ❑ Yes   ❑ Average   ❑ No
Quick service: ❑ Yes   ❑ Average   ❑ Poor
Accuracy: ❑ Good   ❑ Average   ❑ Poor

Ambiance: ❑ Beautiful   ❑ Romantic
    ❑ Average   ❑ Disappointing

Cleanliness Restrooms: ❑ Good   ❑ Average   ❑ Poor
Cleanliness overall: ❑ Good   ❑ Average   ❑ Poor

Drinks ordered: Meals ordered:

Quality overall: ❑ Good   ❑ Average   ❑ Poor

Value for Money: ❑ Overpriced   ❑ OK   ❑ Great

Shall we go again?   ❑ Yes   ❑ No

Memories

Restaurant:
Date:
Time:

Occasion: ❑ Date Night   ❑ Birthday
         ❑

In the company of:

Server name:

Warm welcome: ❑ Yes   ❑ Average   ❑ No
Quick service: ❑ Yes   ❑ Average   ❑ Poor
Accuracy: ❑ Good   ❑ Average   ❑ Poor

Ambiance: ❑ Beautiful   ❑ Romantic
                ❑ Average   ❑ Disappointing

Cleanliness Restrooms: ❑ Good   ❑ Average   ❑ Poor
Cleanliness overall: ❑ Good   ❑ Average   ❑ Poor

Drinks ordered: Meals ordered:

Quality overall: ❑ Good   ❑ Average   ❑ Poor

Value for Money: ❑ Overpriced   ❑ OK   ❑ Great

Shall we go again?   ❑ Yes   ❑ No

Memories

Restaurant:
Date:
Time:

Occasion: ❑ Date Night   ❑ Birthday
❑

In the company of:

Server name:

Warm welcome: ❑ Yes   ❑ Average   ❑ No
Quick service: ❑ Yes   ❑ Average   ❑ Poor
Accuracy: ❑ Good   ❑ Average   ❑ Poor

Ambiance: ❑ Beautiful   ❑ Romantic
❑ Average   ❑ Disappointing

Cleanliness Restrooms: ❑ Good   ❑ Average   ❑ Poor
Cleanliness overall: ❑ Good   ❑ Average   ❑ Poor

Drinks ordered: Meals ordered:

Quality overall: ❑ Good   ❑ Average   ❑ Poor

Value for Money: ❑ Overpriced   ❑ OK   ❑ Great

Shall we go again?   ❑ Yes   ❑ No

Memories

Restaurant:
Date:
Time:

Occasion: ❑ Date Night   ❑ Birthday
              ❑

In the company of:

Server name:

Warm welcome: ❑ Yes   ❑ Average   ❑ No
Quick service: ❑ Yes   ❑ Average   ❑ Poor
Accuracy: ❑ Good   ❑ Average   ❑ Poor

Ambiance: ❑ Beautiful   ❑ Romantic
                ❑ Average   ❑ Disappointing

Cleanliness Restrooms: ❑ Good   ❑ Average   ❑ Poor
Cleanliness overall: ❑ Good   ❑ Average   ❑ Poor

Drinks ordered: Meals ordered:

Quality overall: ❑ Good   ❑ Average   ❑ Poor

Value for Money: ❑ Overpriced   ❑ OK   ❑ Great

Shall we go again?   ❑ Yes   ❑ No

Memories

Pictures Stories Sketches Drawings

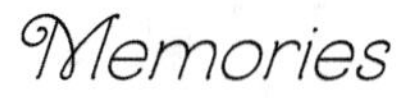

Restaurant:

Date:

Time:

Occasion: ☐ Date Night ☐ Birthday
☐

In the company of:

Server name:

Warm welcome: ☐ Yes ☐ Average ☐ No
Quick service: ☐ Yes ☐ Average ☐ Poor
Accuracy: ☐ Good ☐ Average ☐ Poor

Ambiance: ☐ Beautiful ☐ Romantic
☐ Average ☐ Disappointing

Cleanliness Restrooms: ☐ Good ☐ Average ☐ Poor
Cleanliness overall: ☐ Good ☐ Average ☐ Poor

Drinks ordered: Meals ordered:

Quality overall: ☐ Good ☐ Average ☐ Poor

Value for Money: ☐ Overpriced ☐ OK ☐ Great

Shall we go again? ☐ Yes ☐ No

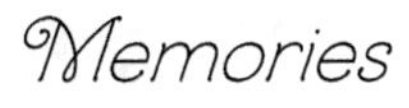

Memories

Restaurant:
Date:
Time:

Occasion: ❑ Date Night   ❑ Birthday
           ❑

In the company of:

Server name:

Warm welcome: ❑ Yes   ❑ Average   ❑ No
Quick service: ❑ Yes   ❑ Average   ❑ Poor
Accuracy: ❑ Good   ❑ Average   ❑ Poor

Ambiance: ❑ Beautiful   ❑ Romantic
            ❑ Average   ❑ Disappointing

Cleanliness Restrooms: ❑ Good   ❑ Average   ❑ Poor
Cleanliness overall: ❑ Good   ❑ Average   ❑ Poor

Drinks ordered: Meals ordered:

Quality overall: ❑ Good   ❑ Average   ❑ Poor

Value for Money: ❑ Overpriced   ❑ OK   ❑ Great

Shall we go again?   ❑ Yes   ❑ No

Memories

Restaurant:

Date:

Time:

Occasion: ❏ Date Night   ❏ Birthday
❏

In the company of:

Server name:

Warm welcome: ❏ Yes   ❏ Average   ❏ No
Quick service: ❏ Yes   ❏ Average   ❏ Poor
Accuracy: ❏ Good   ❏ Average   ❏ Poor

Ambiance: ❏ Beautiful   ❏ Romantic
❏ Average   ❏ Disappointing

Cleanliness Restrooms: ❏ Good   ❏ Average   ❏ Poor
Cleanliness overall: ❏ Good   ❏ Average   ❏ Poor

Drinks ordered: Meals ordered:

Quality overall: ❏ Good   ❏ Average   ❏ Poor

Value for Money: ❏ Overpriced   ❏ OK   ❏ Great

Shall we go again?   ❏ Yes   ❏ No

Memories

Restaurant:
Date:
Time:

Occasion: ❑ Date Night ❑ Birthday
❑

In the company of:

Server name:

Warm welcome: ❑ Yes ❑ Average ❑ No
Quick service: ❑ Yes ❑ Average ❑ Poor
Accuracy: ❑ Good ❑ Average ❑ Poor

Ambiance: ❑ Beautiful ❑ Romantic
❑ Average ❑ Disappointing

Cleanliness Restrooms: ❑ Good ❑ Average ❑ Poor
Cleanliness overall: ❑ Good ❑ Average ❑ Poor

Drinks ordered: Meals ordered:

Quality overall: ❑ Good ❑ Average ❑ Poor

Value for Money: ❑ Overpriced ❑ OK ❑ Great

Shall we go again? ❑ Yes ❑ No

Memories

Restaurant:
Date:
Time:

Occasion: ❑ Date Night   ❑ Birthday
           ❑

In the company of:

Server name:

Warm welcome: ❑ Yes   ❑ Average   ❑ No
Quick service: ❑ Yes   ❑ Average   ❑ Poor
Accuracy: ❑ Good   ❑ Average   ❑ Poor

Ambiance: ❑ Beautiful   ❑ Romantic
           ❑ Average   ❑ Disappointing

Cleanliness Restrooms: ❑ Good   ❑ Average   ❑ Poor
Cleanliness overall: ❑ Good   ❑ Average   ❑ Poor

Drinks ordered: Meals ordered:

Quality overall: ❑ Good   ❑ Average   ❑ Poor

Value for Money: ❑ Overpriced   ❑ OK   ❑ Great

Shall we go again?   ❑ Yes   ❑ No

Memories

Restaurant:
Date:
Time:

Occasion: ❑ Date Night   ❑ Birthday
             ❑

In the company of:

Server name:

Warm welcome: ❑ Yes   ❑ Average   ❑ No
Quick service: ❑ Yes   ❑ Average   ❑ Poor
Accuracy: ❑ Good   ❑ Average   ❑ Poor

Ambiance: ❑ Beautiful   ❑ Romantic
             ❑ Average   ❑ Disappointing

Cleanliness Restrooms: ❑ Good   ❑ Average   ❑ Poor
Cleanliness overall: ❑ Good   ❑ Average   ❑ Poor

Drinks ordered: Meals ordered:

Quality overall: ❑ Good   ❑ Average   ❑ Poor

Value for Money: ❑ Overpriced   ❑ OK   ❑ Great

Shall we go again?   ❑ Yes   ❑ No

Memories

Restaurant:

Date:

Time:

Occasion: ❑ Date Night   ❑ Birthday
           ❑

In the company of:

Server name:

Warm welcome: ❑ Yes   ❑ Average   ❑ No
Quick service: ❑ Yes   ❑ Average   ❑ Poor
Accuracy: ❑ Good   ❑ Average   ❑ Poor

Ambiance: ❑ Beautiful   ❑ Romantic
           ❑ Average   ❑ Disappointing

Cleanliness Restrooms: ❑ Good   ❑ Average   ❑ Poor
Cleanliness overall: ❑ Good   ❑ Average   ❑ Poor

Drinks ordered: Meals ordered:

Quality overall: ❑ Good   ❑ Average   ❑ Poor

Value for Money: ❑ Overpriced   ❑ OK   ❑ Great

Shall we go again?   ❑ Yes   ❑ No

Memories

Restaurant:
Date:
Time:

Occasion: ❑ Date Night   ❑ Birthday
❑

In the company of:

Server name:

Warm welcome: ❑ Yes   ❑ Average   ❑ No
Quick service: ❑ Yes   ❑ Average   ❑ Poor
Accuracy: ❑ Good   ❑ Average   ❑ Poor

Ambiance: ❑ Beautiful   ❑ Romantic
❑ Average   ❑ Disappointing

Cleanliness Restrooms: ❑ Good   ❑ Average   ❑ Poor
Cleanliness overall: ❑ Good   ❑ Average   ❑ Poor

Drinks ordered: Meals ordered:

Quality overall: ❑ Good   ❑ Average   ❑ Poor

Value for Money: ❑ Overpriced   ❑ OK   ❑ Great

Shall we go again?   ❑ Yes   ❑ No

Memories

Restaurant:
Date:
Time:

Occasion: ❑ Date Night ❑ Birthday
❑

In the company of:

Server name:

Warm welcome: ❑ Yes ❑ Average ❑ No
Quick service: ❑ Yes ❑ Average ❑ Poor
Accuracy: ❑ Good ❑ Average ❑ Poor

Ambiance: ❑ Beautiful ❑ Romantic
❑ Average ❑ Disappointing

Cleanliness Restrooms: ❑ Good ❑ Average ❑ Poor
Cleanliness overall: ❑ Good ❑ Average ❑ Poor

Drinks ordered: Meals ordered:

Quality overall: ❑ Good ❑ Average ❑ Poor

Value for Money: ❑ Overpriced ❑ OK ❑ Great

Shall we go again? ❑ Yes ❑ No

Memories

Restaurant:
Date:
Time:

Occasion: ❏ Date Night   ❏ Birthday
                       ❏

In the company of:

Server name:

Warm welcome: ❏ Yes   ❏ Average   ❏ No
Quick service: ❏ Yes   ❏ Average   ❏ Poor
Accuracy: ❏ Good   ❏ Average   ❏ Poor

Ambiance: ❏ Beautiful   ❏ Romantic
                       ❏ Average   ❏ Disappointing

Cleanliness Restrooms: ❏ Good   ❏ Average   ❏ Poor
Cleanliness overall: ❏ Good   ❏ Average   ❏ Poor

Drinks ordered: Meals ordered:

Quality overall: ❏ Good   ❏ Average   ❏ Poor

Value for Money: ❏ Overpriced   ❏ OK   ❏ Great

Shall we go again?   ❏ Yes   ❏ No

Memories

Restaurant:
Date:
Time:

Occasion: ❑ Date Night   ❑ Birthday
                   ❑

In the company of:

Server name:

Warm welcome: ❑ Yes   ❑ Average   ❑ No
Quick service: ❑ Yes   ❑ Average   ❑ Poor
Accuracy: ❑ Good   ❑ Average   ❑ Poor

Ambiance: ❑ Beautiful   ❑ Romantic
                   ❑ Average   ❑ Disappointing

Cleanliness Restrooms: ❑ Good   ❑ Average   ❑ Poor
Cleanliness overall: ❑ Good   ❑ Average   ❑ Poor

Drinks ordered: Meals ordered:

Quality overall: ❑ Good   ❑ Average   ❑ Poor

Value for Money: ❑ Overpriced   ❑ OK   ❑ Great

Shall we go again?   ❑ Yes   ❑ No

Memories

Restaurant:

Date:

Time:

Occasion: ❏ Date Night   ❏ Birthday
           ❏

In the company of:

Server name:

Warm welcome: ❏ Yes   ❏ Average   ❏ No
Quick service: ❏ Yes   ❏ Average   ❏ Poor
Accuracy: ❏ Good   ❏ Average   ❏ Poor

Ambiance: ❏ Beautiful   ❏ Romantic
           ❏ Average   ❏ Disappointing

Cleanliness Restrooms: ❏ Good   ❏ Average   ❏ Poor
Cleanliness overall: ❏ Good   ❏ Average   ❏ Poor

Drinks ordered: Meals ordered:

Quality overall: ❏ Good   ❏ Average   ❏ Poor

Value for Money: ❏ Overpriced   ❏ OK   ❏ Great

Shall we go again?   ❏ Yes   ❏ No

Memories

Restaurant:

Date:

Time:

Occasion: ❑ Date Night   ❑ Birthday
           ❑

In the company of:

Server name:

Warm welcome: ❑ Yes   ❑ Average   ❑ No
Quick service: ❑ Yes   ❑ Average   ❑ Poor
Accuracy: ❑ Good   ❑ Average   ❑ Poor

Ambiance: ❑ Beautiful   ❑ Romantic
           ❑ Average   ❑ Disappointing

Cleanliness Restrooms: ❑ Good   ❑ Average   ❑ Poor
Cleanliness overall: ❑ Good   ❑ Average   ❑ Poor

Drinks ordered: Meals ordered:

Quality overall: ❑ Good   ❑ Average   ❑ Poor

Value for Money: ❑ Overpriced   ❑ OK   ❑ Great

Shall we go again?   ❑ Yes   ❑ No

Restaurant:
Date:
Time:

Occasion: □ Date Night   □ Birthday
           □

In the company of:

Server name:

Warm welcome: □ Yes   □ Average   □ No
Quick service: □ Yes   □ Average   □ Poor
Accuracy: □ Good   □ Average   □ Poor

Ambiance: □ Beautiful   □ Romantic
                 □ Average   □ Disappointing

Cleanliness Restrooms: □ Good   □ Average   □ Poor
Cleanliness overall: □ Good   □ Average   □ Poor

Drinks ordered: Meals ordered:

Quality overall: □ Good   □ Average   □ Poor

Value for Money: □ Overpriced   □ OK   □ Great

Shall we go again?   □ Yes   □ No

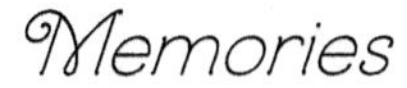

Memories

Restaurant:
Date:
Time:

Occasion: ❏ Date Night ❏ Birthday
❏

In the company of:

Server name:

Warm welcome: ❏ Yes ❏ Average ❏ No
Quick service: ❏ Yes ❏ Average ❏ Poor
Accuracy: ❏ Good ❏ Average ❏ Poor

Ambiance: ❏ Beautiful ❏ Romantic
❏ Average ❏ Disappointing

Cleanliness Restrooms: ❏ Good ❏ Average ❏ Poor
Cleanliness overall: ❏ Good ❏ Average ❏ Poor

Drinks ordered: Meals ordered:

Quality overall: ❏ Good ❏ Average ❏ Poor

Value for Money: ❏ Overpriced ❏ OK ❏ Great

Shall we go again? ❏ Yes ❏ No

Memories

Restaurant:
Date:
Time:

Occasion: ❑ Date Night   ❑ Birthday
    ❑

In the company of:

Server name:

Warm welcome: ❑ Yes   ❑ Average   ❑ No
Quick service: ❑ Yes   ❑ Average   ❑ Poor
Accuracy: ❑ Good   ❑ Average   ❑ Poor

Ambiance: ❑ Beautiful   ❑ Romantic
    ❑ Average   ❑ Disappointing

Cleanliness Restrooms: ❑ Good   ❑ Average   ❑ Poor
Cleanliness overall: ❑ Good   ❑ Average   ❑ Poor

Drinks ordered: Meals ordered:

Quality overall: ❑ Good   ❑ Average   ❑ Poor

Value for Money: ❑ Overpriced   ❑ OK   ❑ Great

Shall we go again?   ❑ Yes ❑ No

Memories

Restaurant:

Date:

Time:

Occasion:
☐ Date Night   ☐ Birthday
☐

In the company of:

Server name:

Warm welcome: ☐ Yes   ☐ Average   ☐ No
Quick service: ☐ Yes   ☐ Average   ☐ Poor
Accuracy: ☐ Good   ☐ Average   ☐ Poor

Ambiance: ☐ Beautiful   ☐ Romantic
     ☐ Average   ☐ Disappointing

Cleanliness Restrooms: ☐ Good   ☐ Average   ☐ Poor
Cleanliness overall: ☐ Good   ☐ Average   ☐ Poor

Drinks ordered: Meals ordered:

Quality overall: ☐ Good   ☐ Average   ☐ Poor

Value for Money: ☐ Overpriced   ☐ OK   ☐ Great

Shall we go again?   ☐ Yes   ☐ No

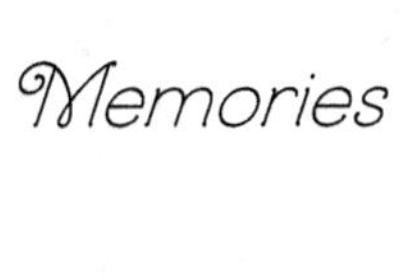

Memories

Restaurant:

Date:

Time:

Occasion: ❑ Date Night   ❑ Birthday
              ❑

In the company of:

Server name:

Warm welcome: ❑ Yes   ❑ Average   ❑ No
Quick service: ❑ Yes   ❑ Average   ❑ Poor
Accuracy: ❑ Good   ❑ Average   ❑ Poor

Ambiance: ❑ Beautiful   ❑ Romantic
                         ❑ Average   ❑ Disappointing

Cleanliness Restrooms: ❑ Good   ❑ Average   ❑ Poor
Cleanliness overall: ❑ Good   ❑ Average   ❑ Poor

Drinks ordered: Meals ordered:

Quality overall: ❑ Good   ❑ Average   ❑ Poor

Value for Money: ❑ Overpriced   ❑ OK   ❑ Great

Shall we go again?   ❑ Yes   ❑ No

Restaurant:
Date:
Time:

Occasion: ❑ Date Night ❑ Birthday
❑

In the company of:

Server name:

Warm welcome: ❑ Yes ❑ Average ❑ No
Quick service: ❑ Yes ❑ Average ❑ Poor
Accuracy: ❑ Good ❑ Average ❑ Poor

Ambiance: ❑ Beautiful ❑ Romantic
❑ Average ❑ Disappointing

Cleanliness Restrooms: ❑ Good ❑ Average ❑ Poor
Cleanliness overall: ❑ Good ❑ Average ❑ Poor

Drinks ordered: Meals ordered:

Quality overall: ❑ Good ❑ Average ❑ Poor

Value for Money: ❑ Overpriced ❑ OK ❑ Great

Shall we go again? ❑ Yes ❑ No

Memories

Restaurant:
Date:
Time:

Occasion: ❑ Date Night   ❑ Birthday
❑

In the company of:

Server name:

Warm welcome: ❑ Yes   ❑ Average   ❑ No
Quick service: ❑ Yes   ❑ Average   ❑ Poor
Accuracy: ❑ Good   ❑ Average   ❑ Poor

Ambiance: ❑ Beautiful   ❑ Romantic
❑ Average   ❑ Disappointing

Cleanliness Restrooms: ❑ Good   ❑ Average   ❑ Poor
Cleanliness overall: ❑ Good   ❑ Average   ❑ Poor

Drinks ordered: Meals ordered:

Quality overall: ❑ Good   ❑ Average   ❑ Poor

Value for Money: ❑ Overpriced   ❑ OK   ❑ Great

Shall we go again?   ❑ Yes   ❑ No

Memories

Restaurant:
Date:
Time:

Occasion: ❏ Date Night   ❏ Birthday
                 ❏

In the company of:

Server name:

Warm welcome: ❏ Yes   ❏ Average   ❏ No
Quick service: ❏ Yes   ❏ Average   ❏ Poor
Accuracy: ❏ Good   ❏ Average   ❏ Poor

Ambiance: ❏ Beautiful   ❏ Romantic
                       ❏ Average   ❏ Disappointing

Cleanliness Restrooms: ❏ Good   ❏ Average   ❏ Poor
Cleanliness overall: ❏ Good   ❏ Average   ❏ Poor

Drinks ordered: Meals ordered:

Quality overall: ❏ Good   ❏ Average   ❏ Poor

Value for Money: ❏ Overpriced   ❏ OK   ❏ Great

Shall we go again?   ❏ Yes   ❏ No

Restaurant:
Date:
Time:

Occasion: ❏ Date Night ❏ Birthday
❏

In the company of:

Server name:

Warm welcome: ❏ Yes ❏ Average ❏ No
Quick service: ❏ Yes ❏ Average ❏ Poor
Accuracy: ❏ Good ❏ Average ❏ Poor

Ambiance: ❏ Beautiful ❏ Romantic
❏ Average ❏ Disappointing

Cleanliness Restrooms: ❏ Good ❏ Average ❏ Poor
Cleanliness overall: ❏ Good ❏ Average ❏ Poor

Drinks ordered: Meals ordered:

Quality overall: ❏ Good ❏ Average ❏ Poor

Value for Money: ❏ Overpriced ❏ OK ❏ Great

Shall we go again? ❏ Yes ❏ No

Memories

Restaurant:

Date:

Time:

Occasion: ❏ Date Night ❏ Birthday
❏

In the company of:

Server name:

Warm welcome: ❏ Yes ❏ Average ❏ No
Quick service: ❏ Yes ❏ Average ❏ Poor
Accuracy: ❏ Good ❏ Average ❏ Poor

Ambiance: ❏ Beautiful ❏ Romantic
❏ Average ❏ Disappointing

Cleanliness Restrooms: ❏ Good ❏ Average ❏ Poor
Cleanliness overall: ❏ Good ❏ Average ❏ Poor

Drinks ordered: Meals ordered:

Quality overall: ❏ Good ❏ Average ❏ Poor

Value for Money: ❏ Overpriced ❏ OK ❏ Great

Shall we go again? ❏ Yes ❏ No

Restaurant:

Date:

Time:

Occasion: ❑ Date Night   ❑ Birthday
           ❑

In the company of:

Server name:

Warm welcome: ❑ Yes   ❑ Average   ❑ No
Quick service: ❑ Yes   ❑ Average   ❑ Poor
Accuracy: ❑ Good   ❑ Average   ❑ Poor

Ambiance: ❑ Beautiful   ❑ Romantic
           ❑ Average   ❑ Disappointing

Cleanliness Restrooms: ❑ Good   ❑ Average   ❑ Poor
Cleanliness overall: ❑ Good   ❑ Average   ❑ Poor

Drinks ordered: Meals ordered:

Quality overall: ❑ Good   ❑ Average   ❑ Poor

Value for Money: ❑ Overpriced   ❑ OK   ❑ Great

Shall we go again?   ❑ Yes   ❑ No

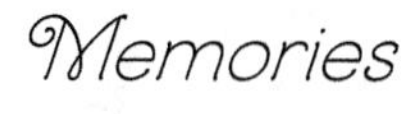

Memories

Restaurant:
Date:
Time:

Occasion: ❑ Date Night   ❑ Birthday
❑

In the company of:

Server name:

Warm welcome: ❑ Yes   ❑ Average   ❑ No
Quick service: ❑ Yes   ❑ Average   ❑ Poor
Accuracy: ❑ Good   ❑ Average   ❑ Poor

Ambiance: ❑ Beautiful   ❑ Romantic
❑ Average   ❑ Disappointing

Cleanliness Restrooms: ❑ Good   ❑ Average   ❑ Poor
Cleanliness overall: ❑ Good   ❑ Average   ❑ Poor

Drinks ordered: Meals ordered:

Quality overall: ❑ Good   ❑ Average   ❑ Poor

Value for Money: ❑ Overpriced   ❑ OK   ❑ Great

Shall we go again?   ❑ Yes   ❑ No

Memories

Restaurant:
Date:
Time:

Occasion: ❏ Date Night   ❏ Birthday
              ❏

In the company of:

Server name:

Warm welcome: ❏ Yes   ❏ Average   ❏ No
Quick service: ❏ Yes   ❏ Average   ❏ Poor
Accuracy: ❏ Good   ❏ Average   ❏ Poor

Ambiance: ❏ Beautiful   ❏ Romantic
                  ❏ Average   ❏ Disappointing

Cleanliness Restrooms: ❏ Good   ❏ Average   ❏ Poor
Cleanliness overall: ❏ Good   ❏ Average   ❏ Poor

Drinks ordered: Meals ordered:

Quality overall: ❏ Good   ❏ Average   ❏ Poor

Value for Money: ❏ Overpriced   ❏ OK   ❏ Great

Shall we go again?   ❏ Yes   ❏ No

Memories

Restaurant:
Date:
Time:

Occasion: ❑ Date Night ❑ Birthday
❑

In the company of:

Server name:

Warm welcome: ❑ Yes ❑ Average ❑ No
Quick service: ❑ Yes ❑ Average ❑ Poor
Accuracy: ❑ Good ❑ Average ❑ Poor

Ambiance: ❑ Beautiful ❑ Romantic
❑ Average ❑ Disappointing

Cleanliness Restrooms: ❑ Good ❑ Average ❑ Poor
Cleanliness overall: ❑ Good ❑ Average ❑ Poor

Drinks ordered: Meals ordered:

Quality overall: ❑ Good ❑ Average ❑ Poor

Value for Money: ❑ Overpriced ❑ OK ❑ Great

Shall we go again? ❑ Yes ❑ No

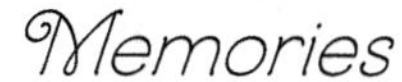

Memories

Restaurant:
Date:
Time:

Occasion: ❑ Date Night   ❑ Birthday
❑

In the company of:

Server name:

Warm welcome: ❑ Yes   ❑ Average   ❑ No
Quick service: ❑ Yes   ❑ Average   ❑ Poor
Accuracy: ❑ Good   ❑ Average   ❑ Poor

Ambiance: ❑ Beautiful   ❑ Romantic
❑ Average   ❑ Disappointing

Cleanliness Restrooms: ❑ Good   ❑ Average   ❑ Poor
Cleanliness overall: ❑ Good   ❑ Average   ❑ Poor

Drinks ordered: Meals ordered:

Quality overall: ❑ Good   ❑ Average   ❑ Poor

Value for Money: ❑ Overpriced   ❑ OK   ❑ Great

Shall we go again?   ❑ Yes   ❑ No

Memories

Restaurant:
Date:
Time:

Occasion: ☐ Date Night   ☐ Birthday
                               ☐

In the company of:

Server name:

Warm welcome: ☐ Yes   ☐ Average   ☐ No
Quick service: ☐ Yes   ☐ Average   ☐ Poor
Accuracy: ☐ Good   ☐ Average   ☐ Poor

Ambiance: ☐ Beautiful   ☐ Romantic
                     ☐ Average   ☐ Disappointing

Cleanliness Restrooms: ☐ Good   ☐ Average   ☐ Poor
Cleanliness overall: ☐ Good   ☐ Average   ☐ Poor

Drinks ordered: Meals ordered:

Quality overall: ☐ Good   ☐ Average   ☐ Poor

Value for Money: ☐ Overpriced   ☐ OK   ☐ Great

Shall we go again?   ☐ Yes   ☐ No

Memories

Restaurant:
Date:
Time:

Occasion: ❏ Date Night   ❏ Birthday
❏

In the company of:

Server name:

Warm welcome: ❏ Yes   ❏ Average   ❏ No
Quick service: ❏ Yes   ❏ Average   ❏ Poor
Accuracy: ❏ Good   ❏ Average   ❏ Poor

Ambiance: ❏ Beautiful   ❏ Romantic
                     ❏ Average   ❏ Disappointing

Cleanliness Restrooms: ❏ Good   ❏ Average   ❏ Poor
Cleanliness overall: ❏ Good   ❏ Average   ❏ Poor

Drinks ordered: Meals ordered:

Quality overall: ❏ Good   ❏ Average   ❏ Poor

Value for Money: ❏ Overpriced   ❏ OK   ❏ Great

Shall we go again?   ❏ Yes   ❏ No

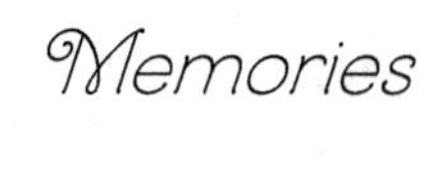

Memories

Restaurant:
Date:
Time:

Occasion: ❑ Date Night   ❑ Birthday
    ❑

In the company of:

Server name:

Warm welcome: ❑ Yes   ❑ Average   ❑ No
Quick service: ❑ Yes   ❑ Average   ❑ Poor
Accuracy: ❑ Good   ❑ Average   ❑ Poor

Ambiance: ❑ Beautiful   ❑ Romantic
    ❑ Average   ❑ Disappointing

Cleanliness Restrooms: ❑ Good   ❑ Average   ❑ Poor
Cleanliness overall: ❑ Good   ❑ Average   ❑ Poor

Drinks ordered: Meals ordered:

Quality overall: ❑ Good   ❑ Average   ❑ Poor

Value for Money: ❑ Overpriced   ❑ OK   ❑ Great

Shall we go again?   ❑ Yes   ❑ No

Memories

Restaurant:
Date:
Time:

Occasion: ❑ Date Night   ❑ Birthday
                        ❑

In the company of:

Server name:

Warm welcome: ❑ Yes   ❑ Average   ❑ No
Quick service: ❑ Yes   ❑ Average   ❑ Poor
Accuracy: ❑ Good   ❑ Average   ❑ Poor

Ambiance: ❑ Beautiful   ❑ Romantic
                        ❑ Average   ❑ Disappointing

Cleanliness Restrooms: ❑ Good   ❑ Average   ❑ Poor
Cleanliness overall: ❑ Good   ❑ Average   ❑ Poor

Drinks ordered: Meals ordered:

Quality overall: ❑ Good   ❑ Average   ❑ Poor

Value for Money: ❑ Overpriced   ❑ OK   ❑ Great

Shall we go again?   ❑ Yes   ❑ No

Memories

Restaurant:
Date:
Time:

Occasion: ❑ Date Night   ❑ Birthday
❑

In the company of:

Server name:

Warm welcome: ❑ Yes   ❑ Average   ❑ No
Quick service: ❑ Yes   ❑ Average   ❑ Poor
Accuracy: ❑ Good   ❑ Average   ❑ Poor

Ambiance: ❑ Beautiful   ❑ Romantic
                 ❑ Average   ❑ Disappointing

Cleanliness Restrooms: ❑ Good   ❑ Average   ❑ Poor
Cleanliness overall: ❑ Good   ❑ Average   ❑ Poor

Drinks ordered: Meals ordered:

Quality overall: ❑ Good   ❑ Average   ❑ Poor

Value for Money: ❑ Overpriced   ❑ OK   ❑ Great

Shall we go again?   ❑ Yes   ❑ No

Memories

Restaurant:
Date:
Time:

Occasion: ❑ Date Night   ❑ Birthday
            ❑

In the company of:

Server name:

Warm welcome: ❑ Yes   ❑ Average   ❑ No
Quick service: ❑ Yes   ❑ Average   ❑ Poor
Accuracy: ❑ Good   ❑ Average   ❑ Poor

Ambiance: ❑ Beautiful   ❑ Romantic
            ❑ Average   ❑ Disappointing

Cleanliness Restrooms: ❑ Good   ❑ Average   ❑ Poor
Cleanliness overall: ❑ Good   ❑ Average   ❑ Poor

Drinks ordered: Meals ordered:

Quality overall: ❑ Good   ❑ Average   ❑ Poor

Value for Money: ❑ Overpriced   ❑ OK   ❑ Great

Shall we go again?   ❑ Yes   ❑ No

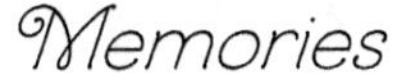

Memories

Restaurant:

Date:

Time:

Occasion: ❑ Date Night   ❑ Birthday
                     ❑

In the company of:

Server name:

Warm welcome: ❑ Yes   ❑ Average   ❑ No
Quick service: ❑ Yes   ❑ Average   ❑ Poor
Accuracy: ❑ Good   ❑ Average   ❑ Poor

Ambiance: ❑ Beautiful   ❑ Romantic
                     ❑ Average   ❑ Disappointing

Cleanliness Restrooms: ❑ Good   ❑ Average   ❑ Poor
Cleanliness overall: ❑ Good   ❑ Average   ❑ Poor

Drinks ordered: Meals ordered:

Quality overall: ❑ Good   ❑ Average   ❑ Poor

Value for Money: ❑ Overpriced   ❑ OK   ❑ Great

Shall we go again?   ❑ Yes   ❑ No

Memories

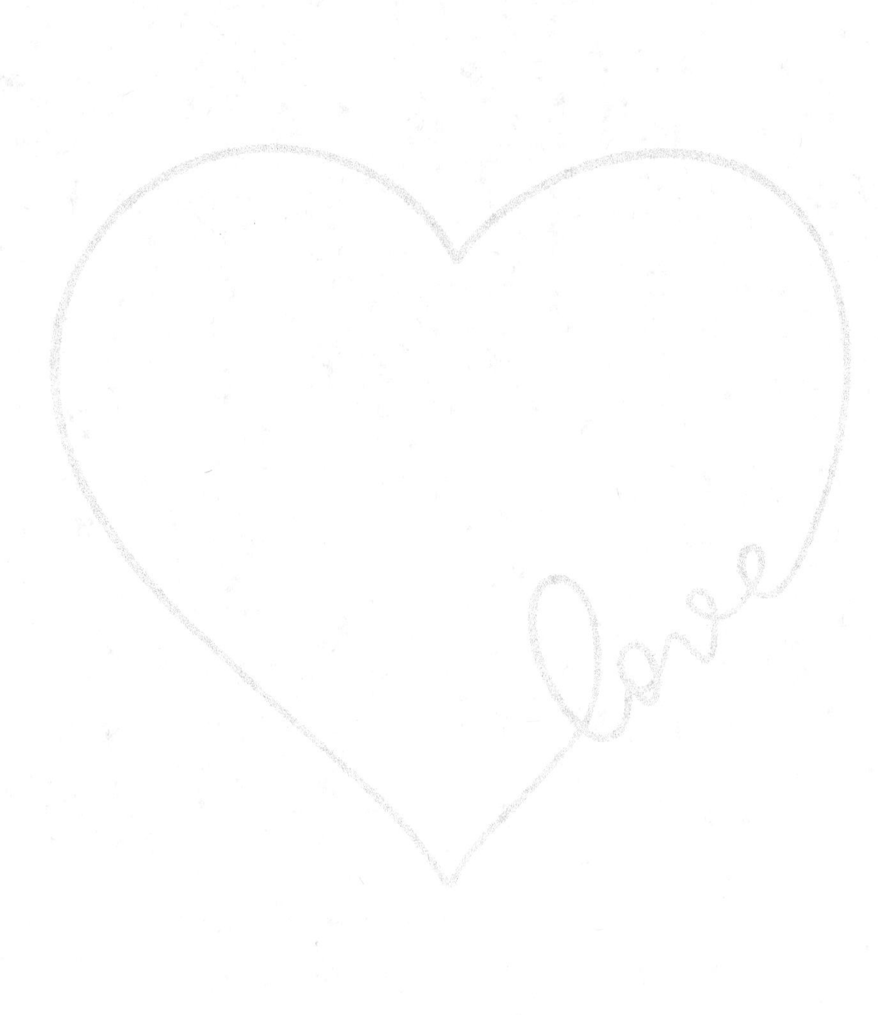